D1826006

Superfood Recipes

The 101 Best Superfood Recipes for Healthy Living and Weight Loss

By

Michelle Brighton

Table of Contents

Introduction

Has your got up and go got up and left? For many of us, the pace of the modern world leaves us exhausted by the end of the day. When I was working in a corporate environment, this was especially true – my "life" consisted of getting up in the morning, having some coffee and cereal and getting to work – always at least an hour before I was meant to so that I could catch up on work before the clients started calling or dropping by.

Lunch was take out quickly ordered from the place around the corner and wolfed down between clients – never even leaving my office. I would often put in ten hours a day at the office and then still take work home. It was when I started considering going in on Sundays as well that I seriously had to reconsider what I had chosen to do for a living.

My lifestyle was nowhere near healthy – exercise consisted of walking to the copier and the only sunlight I usually saw was through my office window. My life consisted of getting up in the morning, having a hurried breakfast, going to work and coming home. I would usually collapse on the couch and veg out in front of the TV before starting the work that I had taken home. (After all, I had sales targets to meet.)

I was overweight, very unhealthy and very unhappy. Looking back, it is amazing that I didn't have a heart attack or stroke at the time.

And what is really sad is that many people reading this will be able to relate – as a society, we are the most technologically advanced that we have ever been but we are also the busiest that we have ever been.

We work hard and we generally do so at the expense of our health and wellness. The good news is that you can start fighting back today – you can start to regain your health and vitality just by making some simple changes in your diet and life.

You work hard and your food should work just as hard – throw out the boring old lettuce salad and swap it out for nutrient dense superfoods that not only taste a lot better but that also pack a huge punch when it comes to nutrients.

This book is packed with 101 of my favorite superfood recipes – each recipe tastes fantastic and is loaded with natural goodness so you can enjoy them without the guilt.

Swap out just one to two meals a week for these recipes – an almost effortless change – and you will find yourself feeling lighter and more vital. Gradually increase the number of meals that include superfoods and you will be super-charging your body, enabling you to make better health choices, cope better with stress and be heathier and more productive overall. Switching over to superfoods is one of the best health decisions that you can make for yourself – and one of the tastiest as well!

Chapter 1:
Salads

A Taste of the East Salad

(Serves 2)

2 tomatoes, diced

1 courgette, peeled and chopped

½ red onion, finely chopped

1 teaspoon cumin

1 teaspoon coriander, finely chopped

½ teaspoon cayenne pepper

1 lemon, juiced

1 tablespoon water

1 tablespoon olive oil

1 teaspoon flaxseed oil

½ teaspoon sesame oil Parsley to serve

Add the tomatoes, courgette and onion in a salad bowl. Mix the spices, lemon juice, water and oils together and pour over the vegetables. Toss and refrigerate for 1 hour. Serve with a few sprigs of parsley.

Rice Salad with a Superfood Boost

(Serves 4)

225 g brown rice

5 mm fresh ginger, sliced finely

285 ml water

3 tablespoon white wine (or more if you like)

50 g raisins

50 g dried apricots, finely chopped up

50 g almonds, roughly chopped

2 medium avocados

Dressing

2 tablespoons extra virgin olive oil

1 tablespoon flaxseed oil

The juice of one lime

1 teaspoon balsamic vinegar

1 teaspoon maple syrup

¼ teaspoon curry powder

¼ teaspoon dry mustard

Make the dressing first by mixing the ingredients well.

Set to one side for at least an hour to allow the flavors to develop properly.

Put the water and ginger in a pot and add the rice.

Add salt to taste and cook until it is just done.

Add your wine, cover with a tight fitting lid and turn the heat to low.

Simmer for 10 minutes before adding the fruit and nuts.

Remove from the heat, cover and leave to sit for 15 minutes.

Add in the dressing and put it in the fridge until nice and cool.

Halve the avocados and remove the pits just before serving.

Serve the rice in the avocado halves.

Cucumber Salad

(Serves 2–4)

2 cucumbers

1 sweet red onion

1 tomato, diced

5 sprigs of parsley, finely chopped up

2 tablespoon freshly picked basil, finely chopped up

2 tablespoon freshly mint, finely chopped up

1 teaspoon flaxseed oil

1 tablespoon extra-virgin olive oil

1 garlic clove, finely chopped up

1 tablespoon balsamic vinegar

Slice the cucumbers and onion thinly and place in a bowl.

Add the chopped tomato and parsley.

Chop the basil and mint and toss them in.

Mix the oils, garlic and vinegar.

Pour over the cucumber and toss together.

Refrigerate for 1 hour and serve.

Avocado and Grapefruit Salad

(Serves 2)

 1 grapefruit

 1 small red onion, finely chopped

1 tablespoon dill, chopped

 1 tablespoon olive oil

1 teaspoon flaxseed oil

The juice of 1 lime

 1 head romaine lettuce

1 ripe avocado

Section the grapefruit into a salad bowl and mix with the chopped onion, dill, oils and lime juice.

Refrigerate for 1 hour.

Chop the lettuce into bite-sized pieces, cube the avocado and add to the grapefruit mix just before serving.

Love Your Veggies

(Serves 2–4)

1 head broccoli, chopped into florets

1 head cauliflower, chopped

2 carrots, sliced

1 red onion, chopped

200g bean sprouts of your choice

Bok choy, roughly chopped

1 yellow bell pepper, sliced

50g raisins

Dressing

1 clove garlic, crushed

¼ teaspoon mustard (optional)

¼ teaspoon parsley stalks, finely chopped

1 tablespoon extra-virgin olive oil

1 teaspoon flaxseed oil 1 teaspoon balsamic vinegar

Crush the garlic, mustard and parsley together, and then mix with the liquid ingredients.

Place all the vegetables and raisins in a salad bowl and toss with the health dressing.

Salad with Israeli Flair

(Serves 4)

1 cucumber, chopped

2 firm and ripe tomatoes, chopped

½ red onion, finely chopped

½ red bell pepper, chopped (optional)

4 sprigs of parsley, chopped

Dressing

1 tablespoon olive oil

The juice of 1 lemon

Salt and pepper

Put the chopped vegetables in a salad bowl.

Peel the cucumber before chopping if it is not organic, but this is not essential.

Chop the onion slightly finer than the other vegetables.

For the dressing, mix the olive oil, lemon juice, salt and pepper together and pour over the vegetables.

Toss and refrigerate.

Dreaming of Africa

(Serves 4)

200g baby kale

2 heads romaine lettuce

1 head butter lettuce

1 fresh pineapple, cut into fingers

2 fresh mangos, cut into strips

1 fresh coconut, cut into strips

1 orange, cut into strips with the skin left on

2 avocados, cut into strips and dipped in lemon juice to prevent browning

The juice of 1 lemon

2 bananas, cut into chunks

2 tablespoons hazelnuts, chopped

225g strawberries, halved

The zest and juice of 3 limes

280ml mayonnaise

150ml whipped cream

2 tablespoons honey

Stem, wash and tear into medium-sized pieces all the greens and place in a salad bowl.

Cut the pineapple into fingers and the mangos, coconut and orange into strips, leaving the skin on the orange.

Cut the avocados into strips and dip them in lemon juice.

Cut the bananas into chunks, dip them in mayonnaise and coat with chopped hazelnuts.

Cut the strawberries in half.

Grate the limes and add the rinds and lime juice to the mayonnaise, cream and honey or agave nectar.

Mix the fruit together with the greens and serve.

Spicy Nigerian Feast

(Serves 4)

2 x 200 g chicken or turkey breasts

225 g large king prawns

Peri-peri sauce

2 large mangos, firm and ripe

2 large avocados, firm and ripe

2 sweet red peppers (pimento)

200 g cherry tomatoes

Rocket salad

½ red onion

Dressing

2 tablespoon olive oil

The juice of 1 lime

1 bunch coriander, chopped

Salt and pepper to taste

Cut the chicken into strips. Marinate the chicken and prawns in peri-peri sauce. Sauté the prawns until cooked. Grill or bake the chicken until cooked through, then set aside to cool.

Cut the mangos and avocados into strips. Chop the red peppers and cut the tomatoes in half. Wash the rocket leaves and place in a bowl. Add all the other ingredients.

Mix the olive oil, lime juice, coriander, salt and pepper. Pour over the salad and toss.

Mango Salad

(Serves 4–6)

2 mangos

½ fresh pineapple 1 orange, juiced

The juice of 1 lemon

 4 avocados (optional)

225g strawberries

Cut the mangos and pineapple into 1 cm cubes and place in a bowl.

Mix the orange and lemon juice together and pour over the mango and pineapple.

Peel, seed and halve the avocados. Place on plates and scoop fruit into each half.

Garnish with strawberries and serve.

Thai Twisted Salad

(Serves 4)

8 lettuce leaves (use different kinds)

2 tablespoons coriander, chopped

2 tablespoons fresh mint, chopped

1 orange, peeled and sectioned

1 can tuna or 1 chicken breast, cooked and shredded

225 g red seedless grapes, halved

½ cucumber, sliced

1 small red onion, thinly sliced

Dressing

Zest of 1 lime

The juice of 2 limes

3 garlic cloves

2 chilies, halved, seeded and cut into pieces

1½ tablespoon fish or soy sauce

1 tablespoon honey

5 tablespoons cashews, chopped

Place half the lettuce in a bowl or on a platter.

Tear the rest of the lettuce leaves into bite sizes and add to the bowl or platter.

Sprinkle the coriander and mint over the lettuce leaves.

Add the orange, tuna or chicken, grapes, cucumber and red onion.

Refrigerate this while you make the dressing.

Grate the lime zest into a blender or food processor.

Add the garlic, chilies, lime juice, fish or soy sauce and honey or agave, and blend until smooth.

Pour the dressing over the salad.

Garnish with cashews and serve.

Indonesian Rice Salad

(Serves 4–6)

250 g brown rice, cooked

5 tablespoons peanut oil, 3 tablespoons sesame oil

1 orange, juiced

1 garlic clove, ¼ teaspoon cayenne pepper

2 tablespoons soy sauce, 1 teaspoon salt

2 tablespoons apple cider vinegar

1 can pineapple, crushed

3 spring onions, chopped, 1 celery stalk, chopped

110 g bean sprouts, 110 g raisins

110 g peanuts, chopped, 110 g cashew pieces

2 tablespoon sesame seeds

1 green pepper, chopped, 1 red pepper, chopped

225 g water chestnut, minced

Mix together the juice, the oil, cayenne pepper, garlic, seasoning, vinegar, pineapple and soy sauce until well combined. Add to the rice.

Stir in the remaining ingredients one at a time so that everything is well-combined. Refrigerate for at least a couple of hours and serve ice cold.

Sesame-Kale Salad

(Serves 2–4)

200 g kale, 1 liter water

Dressing

¼ teaspoon salt (optional)

½ teaspoon honey

1 teaspoon soy sauce

2 tablespoons sesame oil

2 teaspoons sesame seeds

Wash the spinach and remove the stems.

Bring the water with a little salt to a boil. Blanch the spinach in the hot water and then remove to an ice water bath.

Drain the spinach when cool and squeeze it by hand to remove excess moisture. Transfer to a cutting board and chop with a knife.

Mix the salt, honey or agave nectar, soy sauce and sesame oil in a bowl, and set aside. Toss the spinach and dressing in a bowl and garnish with sesame seeds.

Asian Twisted Rice Salad

(Serves 4)

250 g brown or Thai rice, cooked

1 carrot, chopped or shredded

2 spring onions

2 celery stalks, chopped

1 apple, cored and chopped

110 g Chinese peas cut horizontally into 1 cm pieces

50 g peanuts, chopped

Dressing

8 tablespoons olive oil, 2 tablespoons soy sauce

1 lemon or lime, juiced, 1 teaspoon dark sesame oil

1 garlic clove, crushed

Put all the vegetables and fruit in a salad bowl and toss with the cooked rice. Sprinkle with half the nuts, leaving the rest for garnishing.

Whisk the olive oil, soy sauce, lemon juice, sesame oil and garlic in a small bowl. Add half the dressing to the salad and taste. You might require more dressing depending on the type of rice used.

Garnish with the remaining nuts.

Tomato Salad

(Serves 2)

Dressing

4 tablespoons olive or grapeseed oil

2 tablespoons good quality wine vinegar

The juice 1 lime

1 garlic clove, crushed

1 teaspoon Dijon mustard

¼ teaspoon ground cumin

¼ teaspoon salt

¼ teaspoon ground black pepper

5 sprigs fresh mint, chopped

2 large tomatoes, sliced

1 red onion, thinly sliced

½ cucumber, thinly sliced

Make the dressing first by whisking the dressing ingredients together vigorously.

Layer the vegetables and cover with the dressing. Garnish with sprigs of mint. Leave in the refrigerator overnight to allow flavors to develop.

Greek Salad

(Serves 2)

1 head romaine lettuce, torn into bite- sized pieces

1 red onion, sliced

1 cucumber, sliced

4 tomatoes, sliced

Kalamata olives

Feta cheese, crumbled

Dressing

4 tablespoon olive oil

1 lemon, juiced

2 garlic cloves, crushed

1 teaspoon dried oregano

Whisk together the oil, lemon, garlic and oregano, and set aside.

Put all the vegetables in a bowl.

Add the olives and cheese.

Pour the dressing over the salad and toss.

Serve with pita and hummus.

Apple and Kale Salad

(Serves 2)

3 apples, peeled, cored and diced

3 spring onions, chopped

3 celery stalks, chopped

The juice of 2 lemons

4 tablespoons mayonnaise

4 tablespoon tahini

2 tablespoons honey

1 bunch kale, torn into bite-sized pieces

4 tablespoons sesame seeds

Put the apples, onions and celery in a large bowl.

Sprinkle with the juice of 1 lemon to avoid discoloration, and set aside.

In a blender or bowl, blend or whisk the mayonnaise, tahini, honey or agave and the remaining lemon juice until the mixture thickens.

Mix into the salad.

Cover and refrigerate until it is time to serve.

Just before serving, toss in the spinach and garnish with sesame seeds.

Greek Sweet Potato Salad

(Serves 2–4)

4 sweet potatoes

1 red onion, sliced

4 tablespoon olive oil

1 lemon, juiced

2 celery stalks, chopped

Salt and black pepper to taste

5 sprigs parsley, chopped

Boil the potatoes until tender and keep them hot.

Place the onion in a large bowl.

Sprinkle with salt and cold water and allow to stand for 5 minutes. Then drain.

Slice the potatoes and add to the onions.

Add the olive oil, lemon juice and celery, and mix well to absorb the dressing.

Season with salt and pepper and garnish with parsley.

Serve warm.

Grilled Veggie Salad

(Serves 2)

2 large red bell peppers

4 medium tomatoes

2 large red onions

1 small hot pepper

1 can tuna

4 tablespoon feta cheese, crumbled

Dressing

3 tablespoon olive oil

The juice of 1 lemon

1 teaspoon oregano

Salt and black pepper to taste

Grill the peppers, tomatoes and onions in a hot oven at 200°C. Turn over once and grill until soft. Remove from the oven and cool. Remove the seeds from the pepper and chop all the vegetables into small pieces.

Place the vegetables on a serving platter and top with tuna and feta cheese.

Whisk the olive oil, lemon juice, oregano, salt and pepper, and pour over the salad. Serve.

Macedonian Salad

(Serves 4)

¼ head white cabbage

⅛ Head red cabbage

1 green pepper, chopped

1 red pepper, chopped

4 sprigs parsley, chopped

2 celery stalks, chopped

1 carrot

2 tablespoons olive oil

½ lemon, juiced

Salt to taste

Cut the cabbage into thin strips and place in a bowl.

Add the peppers, parsley and celery.

Grate the carrot and add to the bowl.

Sprinkle with olive oil, lemon juice and salt to taste.

Mix well and serve.

Pomegranate and Veggie Salad

(Serves 2–4)

2 green bell peppers, cut into 1 cm cubes

4 large tomatoes, cut into 1 cm cubes

2 red onions, chopped finely

2 cucumbers, peeled and cut into 1 cm cubes

½ pomegranate

Dressing

4 tablespoons olive oil

2 tablespoons white wine vinegar

¼ teaspoon coarse salt and black pepper

Put the vegetables in a bowl.

Mix the olive oil, vinegar, salt and pepper together.

Add the dressing to the salad and toss.

Hold the pomegranate over the salad.

Using a spatula or spoon, release the seeds and juice over the salad.

Refrigerate for 1 hour before serving.

Chapter 2:
Dips & Dressings

Salad Dressings

Basic Superfood Dressing

1 tablespoon extra-virgin olive oil

1 teaspoon flaxseed oil

1 teaspoon balsamic vinegar

1 garlic clove

¼ teaspoon dry mustard

¼ teaspoon parsley, finely chopped

Mash the garlic, mustard and parsley together.

Mix with other ingredients.

Use this dressing with any salad.

Lemony Dressing

4 tablespoon fresh mint, chopped

4 tablespoon fresh parsley, chopped

1 lemon

2 tablespoon olive oil

1 teaspoon flaxseed oil

Mix all ingredients together and use over salad.
Try it with cucumber salad.

Asian Dressing

1 lime

3 garlic cloves

2 fiery chilies, halved, seeded and chopped

1½ tablespoon fish sauce or soy sauce

1 tablespoon honey

Crush the garlic and mix in with all other
ingredients.

Indian Style Dressing

4 tablespoons grapeseed oil

2 tablespoons white wine vinegar

The juice of ½ fresh lime

1 garlic clove

1 teaspoon Dijon mustard

¼ teaspoon ground cumin

¼ teaspoon salt

¼ teaspoon ground black pepper

2 tablespoons mint, chopped

Crush the garlic with the mint and mix in with the other ingredients.

Greek Dressing

3 tablespoons olive oil

1½ tablespoons red or white-wine vinegar

½ teaspoon salt

¼ teaspoon oregano

¼ teaspoon freshly-ground black pepper

Put all ingredients in a small jar, close and shake thoroughly.

Chill before serving.

Italian Dressing

4 tablespoons extra virgin olive oil

2 tablespoons red-wine vinegar

80ml water

½ teaspoon salt

½ teaspoon black pepper

1 teaspoon oregano

1 teaspoon garlic powder or 1 garlic clove, crushed

Put all ingredients in a jar and shake thoroughly.

Great Dips

Red Pepper Dip

3 red peppers

2 tablespoons fresh lemon juice

2 tablespoons fresh parsley

1 tablespoon olive oil

Salt to taste

Cut and deseed the red peppers.

Bake them in the oven on a low temperature for about 20–25 minutes. Then remove the skin.

In a food processor, blend the peppers, lemon juice, parsley, olive oil and salt.

Serve with any veggie sticks such as carrots or cucumbers.

Salsa Dip

5 tomatoes, chopped

1 jalapeno pepper, chopped

1 red bell pepper, chopped

2 tablespoons coriander, finely chopped

2 tablespoons parsley, finely chopped

1 small red onion, finely chopped

2 garlic cloves, crushed

1 teaspoon balsamic vinegar or lemon juice

Mix all ingredients together, chill and serve.

Yellow Split Pea Dip

250g dried yellow split peas, rinsed and drained

¾ teaspoon salt

½ teaspoon black pepper

1 liter water

1 onion, chopped

2 tablespoon extra-virgin oil

1 tomato, finely chopped

1 red bell pepper, finely chopped

1 tablespoon fresh parsley, chopped

Put the split peas with a pinch of salt and black pepper in a saucepan. Pour in enough water to cover the peas by 2½ cm and bring to the boil. Reduce the heat to medium and simmer, uncovered, stirring occasionally and adding more water, a little at a time, if it gets too thick before the peas get soft which takes about an hour.

Mash the peas and allow to cool. Stir in half the onion, oil and remaining salt and pepper. Spread this purée out in a shallow bowl. In a small bowl, mix the remaining onion, tomato, red pepper and parsley. Sprinkle over the purée

Chapter 3:

Healthy and Substantial Soups

Mixed Vegetable Soup

(Serves 2–4)

1 tablespoon olive oil

2½ cm ginger, crushed

1 garlic clove, crushed

2 carrots, finely chopped

1 head cauliflower, chopped

50g broccoli, chopped

1 red pepper, chopped

½ head cabbage, finely chopped

5 green beans, chopped

600 ml water

2 potatoes, chopped

½ teaspoon soy sauce

¼ teaspoon red chili powder

1 medium onion, chopped

½ teaspoon honey

Heat the oil in a saucepan.

Add the ginger and garlic, and cook for 1 minute.

Add all the vegetables except the potatoes and onion.

Add salt and stir-fry for 4–5 minutes or until the vegetables are cooked.

Pour in the water and bring to the boil.

Add the potatoes, soy sauce and chili.

Boil until the soup becomes thick and transparent.

Finally, add the chopped onion and honey and boil for another 2–3 minutes.

Serve hot.

Saffron Flavored Soup

(Serves 4–6)

 4 tablespoons olive oil

2 medium onions, chopped

2 fennel bulbs, chopped

3 garlic cloves, crushed

1 teaspoon saffron

1 tablespoon boiling water

125 ml white wine

50 g fresh basil, shredded

1 kg tomatoes, finely chopped

450 ml water

 Salt and black pepper to taste

100g shredded basil to garnish

Heat the oil in a large pot.

Sauté the onions, fennel and garlic over a medium heat for about 10 minutes.

Crumble and soak the saffron in 1 tablespoon of boiling water for 5 minutes.

Pour the wine and soaked saffron, into the onions, fennel and garlic, then stir in 50 g of basil.

Bring to a boil, then reduce the heat and simmer for a minute or two.

Add the chopped tomatoes and water.

Bring to a boil, reduce the heat and simmer for about 30 minutes, partially covered.

Before serving, add salt and black pepper to taste, then stir in the basil.

Serve hot.

Shrimp Soup

(Serves 4)

2 tablespoons olive oil

1 onion, coarsely chopped

2 garlic cloves, crushed

2 cans of tomatoes, deseeded and chopped, reserving juice

4 Portobello mushrooms, sliced

5 parsley sprigs, chopped

2 celery stalks, chopped

1 bay leaf

½ teaspoon black pepper

½ teaspoon cayenne pepper

1 liter fish stock

200 ml dry white wine

2 potatoes

450g raw shrimps, peeled

½ teaspoon salt

In a large saucepan, sauté the onion and garlic in oil for about 5 minutes.

Mix in the tomatoes, mushrooms, parsley, celery, bay leaf, black pepper and cayenne pepper.

Lower the heat and cook for about 10–15 minutes.

Slowly pour in the fish stock and wine.

Stir through and bring to the boil. When the soup is boiling, grate in the potatoes and allow the mixture to thicken.

Reduce the heat and stir in the peeled shrimps.

Simmer for 10–15 minutes.

Add salt to taste and serve.

Shrimp & Sea Bass Soup with Orzo

(Serves 4–6)

2 garlic cloves, sliced

1 teaspoon cumin

1 teaspoon paprika

½ teaspoon salt

½ teaspoon black pepper

4 tablespoons tomato purée

2 tablespoons olive oil

1 medium onion, thinly sliced

1 liter fish stock

450g sea bass cut in chunks

200g shrimps

75g orzo (rice-shaped pasta or any other soup pasta – add more if required)

4 parsley sprigs, chopped

½ each of lemon and lime, sliced thinly

Crush the garlic with the cumin, paprika, salt and pepper in a food processor.

Mix in the tomato purée.

Heat the oil in a large saucepan.

Add the onion and sauté for about 5 minutes.

Add the spice mixture and stir for 3 minutes.

Pour in the fish stock and bring to the boil.

Lower the heat and add the fish and shrimps.

Cook for 10 minutes.

Add the orzo and cook for 10 minutes.

Garnish with parsley and serve with wedges of lime and lemon on the side.

Indian Tomato Soup

(Serves 2)

5 tomatoes deseeded, 2 quartered and 3 chopped

1 garlic clove

550 ml water

2 teaspoons ginger, crushed

50g coriander, chopped

1 deseeded green chili pepper, cut into small pieces

1 teaspoon curry powder

½ teaspoon cumin

½ teaspoon black pepper

2 teaspoons salt

2 teaspoons olive oil

¼ teaspoon black mustard seeds

2 deseeded red chili peppers

Purée the quartered tomatoes with the garlic in a food processor and set aside.

Boil the water in a medium-sized saucepan.

Add the puréed tomatoes, ginger, coriander and green chili.

Turn the heat down and simmer for 3 minutes.

Add the tomato and garlic purée, curry, cumin, black pepper and salt and simmer for 5 minutes.

Put the oil and mustard seed in a small saucepan over a high heat.

Cover and cook until you hear the mustard seeds crackle, which takes about 1–2 minutes.

Add the red chilies and cook uncovered, stirring until they start to brown.

This takes about 60 seconds.

Pour into the soup and stir. Serve hot.

Spicy Tomato Soup

(Serves 4)

2 garlic cloves

1 serrano green chili, seeded

1 onion, chopped coarsely

1 cucumber, diced

2 tablespoons salt

450g tomatoes, firm and ripe

1 tablespoon tamarind paste

225g fresh coriander, chopped

110g fresh mint, chopped

2½ cm ginger, grated 1 teaspoon ground cumin

225ml non-fat plain yoghurt (optional)

1 teaspoon olive oil

2 teaspoons cumin seeds

1 teaspoon yellow mustard seeds 1 teaspoon black mustard seeds

In a food processor, blend the garlic and chili until minced. Add the onion and mince again. Scrape into a large bowl and stir in the cucumber and salt.

Meanwhile, bring 3 liters of water to the boil. Cut an X in the bottom of each tomato and immerse in the boiling water for 30 seconds or until the tomato skin begins to curl.

Rinse under cold running water until cool and remove skins. Chop the tomatoes and add with the juice to the bowl containing the onion mixture.

In a small bowl, mix the tamarind paste with 4 tablespoon of warm water and pour into the tomato mixture. Add the coriander, mint and ginger, and mix.

In a saucepan over a medium heat, stir the cumin for 2 minutes, until fragrant. Add the tomato mixture and 400 ml water, and bring to the boil.

Remove from the heat, cover and chill for at least an hour. Ladle the soup into bowls and top each serving with yoghurt (optional).

In a non-stick pan with a lid, add the oil, cumin and mustard seeds. Set over a high heat until the spices begin to pop. Cover and shake vigorously until the popping subsides, which should take about 1–2 minutes. Spoon the hot seeds over the soup and serve.

Creamy African Soup

(Serves 4)

2 skinless chicken breasts, chopped

1 liter water

2 tablespoons olive oil-based or unsalted butter

3 Granny Smith apples, peeled, cored and chopped

2 celery stalks, chopped

2 carrots, chopped

1 onion, chopped

1 garlic clove, crushed

3 tablespoon curry powder

50g golden raisins

1 sweet potato, diced

110 ml coconut milk

Salt to taste

½ teaspoon cayenne

½ white pepper

Mango chutney to garnish

Put the chicken in a large saucepan with 1 liters of water and bring to the boil.

Remove the chicken when cooked and set aside, reserving the broth.

In a saucepan, heat the oil-based fat or butter over a medium heat until the foam subsides.

Add the apples, celery, carrots, onion and garlic, stirring occasionally until they begin to soften which should take about 10 minutes.

Add the curry powder, chicken and raisins, and cook for about a minute.

Add the diced sweet potato, cook and stir for 2 minutes.

Stir in the chicken broth, cover and simmer for 1 hour. Stir in the coconut milk and salt to taste. Simmer uncovered for 10 minutes.

Add the cayenne and white pepper.

Cool the soup. Then pour into a food processor or blender in batches, and blend until smooth.

Strain the soup into a large bowl and chill for about 2 to 3 hours until cold. Garnish with ½ teaspoon of chutney and serve.

Pea Soup

(Serves 4)

2 onions, chopped

2 garlic cloves, crushed

2½ cm ginger, peeled and grated

1 teaspoon salt

¼ teaspoon cayenne pepper

1 tablespoon garam masala

2 tomatoes, chopped

1 sweet potato, diced

700 ml water

600 g green peas

Sauté the onions and garlic in a saucepan for 5 to 10 minutes.

Add the ginger, salt, cayenne pepper and garam masala and cook for a few minutes, stirring often.

Mix in the tomatoes and sweet potato.

Add 400 ml water and stir.

Bring to the boil.

Reduce the heat, cover and simmer for 5 minutes.

Add half the peas, cover and simmer for 10 minutes.

Remove from the heat and add the remaining water.

Blend in batches in a blender until smooth.

Return to the saucepan.

Add the remaining peas and cook on a medium heat for 3–5 minutes.

Vegetable Soup

(Serves 4–6)

2 onions, chopped

1 garlic clove, crushed

30 ml olive oil

3 carrots, sliced

2 turnips, sliced

2 celery stalks, chopped

4 courgettes, sliced

1 small butternut squash, peeled, deseeded and chopped

2 medium eggplants, peeled and diced

2 tablespoons fresh tarragon or thyme, chopped

1 liter vegetable or chicken stock

Salt and black pepper to taste

Sauté the onions and garlic in oil in a heavy-based saucepan for about 5 minutes.

Add the carrots, turnips, celery, courgettes, butternut squash, eggplants, tarragon or thyme and stock.

Bring to the boil.

Reduce the heat, cover the saucepan and simmer for about 25 minutes or until the vegetables are soft.

Season to taste and serve.

Tomato and Carrot Soup

(Serves 4–6)

1 tablespoon olive oil

1 onion, chopped

2 garlic cloves, chopped

2 carrots, peeled and chopped

500 g tomatoes, skinned and coarsely chopped

1 apple, peeled, cored and chopped

1 bouquet garni

1 bay leaf

1 liter vegetable or chicken stock

Salt and freshly ground black pepper to taste

60 ml cream to garnish (optional)

Heat the oil in a large saucepan.

Add the onion and garlic and sauté for 10 minutes.

Add the carrots and stir over a low heat until all the oil has been absorbed.

Add the tomatoes, apple, bouquet garni, bay leaf and stock.

Season with salt and black pepper, and bring to the boil.

Cover the saucepan and simmer for 45 minutes.

Remove and discard the bouquet garni.

Pour the soup into a blender.

Return the soup to the saucepan, heat through and adjust the seasoning.

Pour into individual bowls, garnish with 1 tablespoon of cream (optional) and serve.

Sweet Potato Soup

(Serves 4)

1 tablespoon olive oil   2 onions, chopped

1 serrano green chili pepper or jalapeno, sliced thinly

1 liter vegetable or chicken stock

3 sweet potatoes, peeled and chopped

2½ cm ginger, grated

1 teaspoon thyme

Salt and black pepper to taste

4 sausages, sliced thickly (optional)

Juice of 1 lemon

Sauté the onions in the oil in a saucepan until transparent.

Add the sliced pepper and stock.

Bring to the boil over a medium heat.

Add the sweet potatoes, ginger and thyme.

Boil then reduce the heat and simmer for 25 minutes, stirring occasionally.

When the potatoes are cooked, pour into a food processor, solids first, and purée.

Season with salt and black pepper to taste.

If you are having the soup hot and meaty, sauté the sausage separately until crisp.

When ready to serve, stir in the lemon juice, then pour the soup into individual bowls, either cold or hot.

Add the sausage, if applicable, and top with lemon curls.

Lentil and Courgette Soup

(Serves 4)

275g dried lentils

1 onion, chopped

4 garlic cloves, crushed

1 liter water

2 potatoes, cut into small pieces

1 teaspoon cumin

1 celery stalk, chopped

2 courgettes, cut into small pieces

Salt and black pepper to taste

2 lemons, cut into wedges to serve on the side

Put the lentils, onion and garlic into a large saucepan.

Add the water, cover and bring to the boil.

Reduce the heat and simmer for 20 minutes.

Stir in the potatoes, cumin, celery and courgettes.

Cover and cook for 15 minutes, until the lentils and potatoes are tender.

Season with salt and black pepper to taste.

When the soup is ready to serve, pour it into soup bowls, sprinkle with lemon juice and serve a lemon wedge with each bowl.

Moroccan Carrot Soup

(Serves 4)

1 liter vegetable or chicken stock 450g carrots, peeled and chopped

1 garlic clove, crushed

⅛ Teaspoon cinnamon

¼ teaspoon cumin

½ teaspoon paprika

½ teaspoon cayenne pepper or hot sauce

Juice of 1 lemon

½ teaspoon honey

½ teaspoon orange flower water

1 tablespoon parsley, chopped

In a medium saucepan, boil the stock.

Add the carrots and garlic.

Reduce the heat and simmer until the carrots are tender.

Remove half the carrots and set aside.

In a food processor, blend the carrots, garlic and stock, then return to the saucepan.

Mix in the cinnamon, cumin, paprika and cayenne or hot sauce.

Add the remaining carrots to the soup, and simmer for 10 minutes.

When the soup is ready to serve, stir in the lemon juice, honey or agave and orange flower water.

Serve in bowls and sprinkle with parsley.

Shiitake Bok Choy Soup

(Serves 4)

½ onion, chopped

2 carrots, peeled and sliced

10 dried shiitake mushrooms, broken up

700 ml water

2 tablespoon sesame oil

1 teaspoon honey

1 cm ginger, crushed

1 tablespoon soy sauce

½ teaspoon each salt and black pepper

110 g bok choy

Put the onion, carrots and mushrooms into a saucepan and add the water.

Bring to the boil and simmer until the carrots and mushrooms are soft.

Add the sesame oil, honey or agave, ginger and soy sauce. Add salt and black pepper to taste.

Bring back to the boil, then add the bok choy and simmer until it is tender which should take about 3 minutes.

Melon Soup

(Serves 4)

300 ml water

½ teaspoon salt

1 onion, chopped

8 chicken pieces

1 tablespoon ground crayfish

2 tablespoon palm oil

200 g spinach, chopped

125 g ground melon seeds

In a saucepan, add the water, salt, onion and chicken, and bring to the boil for 10 minutes.

Add the ground crayfish and palm oil and simmer for 10 minutes.

Sprinkle over the ground melon seeds and simmer on a low heat for 10–15 minutes, stirring just once.

Add the spinach and cook for an additional 5 minutes or until it has just wilted. If you are using fish, add this last and cook for 10 minutes or until the fish is cooked through.

Chapter 4:
Starters and Vegetables

Asian-style Coleslaw

(Serves 2–4)

½ medium head white cabbage, sliced

½ medium head red cabbage, sliced

1 red pepper, chopped

1 yellow pepper, chopped

3 carrots, peeled and shredded

4 spring onions

½ bunch fresh coriander, chopped

50 g roasted peanuts, chopped

3 tablespoons rice vinegar

1 tablespoon sesame oil

2 tablespoons soy sauce

1 tablespoon honey or agave nectar

1 cm fresh ginger, peeled and minced

1 garlic clove, crushed

1 jalapeno pepper, deseeded and finely chopped

Toss the salad ingredients in a bowl. Mix the vinegar, sesame oil, soy sauce, honey or agave, ginger, garlic and pepper. Mix into the salad.

Bean Cakes

(Serves 6)

250g black-eyed beans

(Bean flour can be used but it's not the best option)

1 onion

1 red chili pepper

2 tablespoon dried ground crayfish

100 g cooked prawns

2 tablespoon grapeseed oil 1 teaspoon salt

3 hard-boiled eggs (optional), cut into chunks

6 foil takeout boxes

Place the beans in a large bowl. Cover with water and soak overnight.

The following day, rub the beans briskly between your palms to remove the skins.

Fill the bowl with water and the skins will float to the top. Discard the skins.

Continue this action until the beans are clean and no skins are left behind – soak them again if necessary.

In a food processor, blend the beans, onion, ground black pepper and 10 ml of water until smooth.

Pour into a bowl. Add the crayfish, prawns, oil and salt and mix thoroughly.

In a large saucepan, add enough water just to fill the base and bring to the boil.

Use the foil boxes as a measuring guide: only half of the box should be submerged in water.

Pour small amounts of the mixture into individual boxes. If you are using eggs, add some into each box.

Cover with the lids, place in the saucepan and steam for an hour until firm.

Serve warm or hot with tomato sauce and salad.

A Fun Green Salad

(Serves 4)

3 avocados (ripe but firm), stone removed and cut into cubes

Juice of ½ lemon

2 tablespoons peanuts, ground

½ teaspoon cinnamon

½ teaspoon paprika

Salt and chili powder to taste

1 bunch romaine lettuce leaves, separated and washed

10 g fresh chives, chopped to garnish

Place the cubed avocado in a bowl and sprinkle with lemon juice. Set aside.

Mix the ground peanuts, cinnamon, paprika, salt and chili powder together thoroughly.

Arrange the individual lettuce leaves on a platter like cups.

Scoop avocado onto each lettuce leaf, sprinkle peanut mixture over the avocado and garnish with chives.

Courgettes with Garlic Cream Sauce

(Serves 4–6)

2 tablespoons unsalted butter

6 garlic cloves, crushed

1 onion, finely chopped

3 leeks, finely chopped

1 teaspoon fresh thyme, chopped

3 medium courgettes, washed and grated

3 medium yellow squash, washed and grated

2½ tablespoon sour cream

½ teaspoon fresh ground black pepper

Melt the butter in a saucepan. Add the garlic, onion and leeks and sauté over a low heat for 5 minutes.

Mix in the thyme, courgettes and squash.

Cook, stirring frequently for 5– 7 minutes or until the courgettes and squash are tender.

Place on a plate, top with sour cream and sprinkle with ground black pepper.

Bok Choy Slaw

(Serves 4)

4 tablespoons rice wine vinegar

1 tablespoon sesame oil

2 teaspoons honey

2 teaspoons Dijon mustard

¼ teaspoon salt

600 g bok choy, washed and thinly sliced

2 carrots, peeled and shredded

2 spring onions, chopped thinly

In a medium bowl, whisk the vinegar, oil, honey, mustard and salt until smooth.

Add the bok choy, carrots and spring onions.

Toss to coat thoroughly with the dressing.

Veggie Stir Fry

(Serves 4)

1 tablespoon grapeseed oil

2 red onions, sliced

150 g mushrooms, sliced

1 head white cabbage or Chinese cabbage, shredded

2 courgettes, chopped

2 tablespoons Szechuan stir-fry sauce

1 teaspoon sesame oil

1 teaspoon agave nectar or honey (optional)

Salt and pepper to taste

Heat the grapeseed oil in a wok or saucepan. Sauté the onions for 2 minutes.

Add the mushrooms and courgettes and cook for 3 minutes. Mix in the cabbage.

Drizzle the stir-fry sauce over the vegetables and sauté until the cabbage is just wilted.

Drizzle with sesame oil and agave or honey (if you are using it for a sweet twist).

Add salt and pepper to taste. Mix thoroughly.

Spicy Vegetables

(Serves 2–4)

2 tablespoons olive oil

2 teaspoons black mustard seeds

2 onions, finely chopped

2 garlic cloves, chopped

1 cm ginger, chopped

½ teaspoon turmeric

½ teaspoon coriander

1 teaspoon ground cumin

¼ teaspoon chili powder

2 carrots, peeled and chopped

2 sweet potatoes, peeled and chopped

2 tomatoes, chopped

250 g green beans, trimmed and cut into small pieces

Salt and pepper to taste

½ teaspoon garam masala

Heat the oil in a heavy saucepan and fry the mustard seeds until they pop.

Add the onions, garlic and ginger. Sauté, stirring continuously for 5 minutes or until the onions are golden.

Add the turmeric, coriander, cumin and chili powder, and sauté for about 30 seconds. Then toss in the vegetables.

Mix until they are thoroughly coated with the spices.

Add salt, pepper and 3 tablespoons of water.

Cover and cook for 15 minutes or until the vegetables are tender.

Stir gently every 5 minutes and add a little more water if necessary.

Sprinkle with garam masala and stir.

Stewed Greens

(Serves 4–6)

600 g collard greens, washed and chopped

200 g spinach, washed

200 g kale

4 tablespoons olive oil

1 onion, chopped

4 tomatoes, chopped

1 green chili pepper, deseeded and finely chopped

Juice of ½ lemon

1 tablespoon plain unbleached flour

225 ml water

½ teaspoon salt and black pepper

Steam the greens in a steamer for about 6 minutes.

If you don't have a steamer, pour water into a saucepan and bring to the boil. Place the greens in a colander and insert into the saucepan. Cover and steam for about 6 minutes.

Heat 2 tablespoon of oil in a frying pan over a medium heat.

Add the onion, tomatoes and pepper.

Mix well and cook for about 5 minutes.

Reduce the heat to low and add the remaining oil.

Whisk the lemon juice, flour and half the water until smooth and well- blended.

Pour into the onion mixture and mix well.

Add the remaining water, cooked greens, salt and pepper to taste and mix well.

Increase the heat to medium, cover and cook for 3 minutes to heat through.

Serve with a main dish such as fish or chicken.

Asparagus and Sun-dried Tomatoes

(Serves 2)

1 tablespoon olive oil

1 teaspoon flaxseed oil

1 teaspoon balsamic vinegar

½ teaspoon cayenne pepper

2 tablespoons sun-dried tomatoes, chopped

15 g parsley, chopped

225 g asparagus

10 g fresh basil, chopped

In a small bowl, mix the oils, vinegar, cayenne, tomatoes and half of the parsley together.

Leave to marinade for 2 hours.

Steam the asparagus for about 6 minutes or until just tender.

Place the asparagus on a plate.

Pour the sauce over, and sprinkle with the remaining parsley and basil.

Baked Tomatoes

(Serves 2–4)

2 tablespoon olive oil

4 large tomatoes, cored and cut into 3 thick slices each

200 g breadcrumbs

20 g fresh basil, chopped

1 teaspoon fresh thyme, chopped

1 teaspoon fresh oregano, chopped

1 garlic clove, chopped

Extra olive oil to drizzle

Preheat the oven to 180°C or Gas Mark 4. Lightly brush half the olive oil on a baking tray.

Arrange the tomato slices, cut side up, in a single layer. Mix the breadcrumbs, remaining oil, half the herbs and garlic. Sprinkle over the tomatoes.

Bake for about 5–7 minutes or until the breadcrumbs are lightly browned.

Place the tomatoes on a serving platter, sprinkle with remaining herbs and drizzle with olive oil.

Warm Bok Choy

(Serves 2–4)

1 onion, chopped

2½ cm ginger, grated

1 tablespoon olive oil

½ teaspoon sesame oil

500 g bok choy, both white and green parts sliced

1 tablespoon rice wine vinegar

1 teaspoon fish sauce

½ teaspoon red pepper, crushed

Salt to taste

100 ml chicken stock

1 tablespoon sesame seeds

In a medium-sized saucepan, sauté the onion and ginger in the oils for 5 minutes.

Add the bok choy, vinegar, fish sauce, pepper, salt and stock.

Mix and sauté for about 8 minutes.

Place on a plate and sprinkle with sesame seeds.

Balsamic Mushrooms

(Serves 2)

½ teaspoon sesame oil

1 onion, chopped

350 g shiitake mushrooms

2 tablespoon sundried tomatoes (optional)

2 tablespoon balsamic vinegar

1 tablespoon red wine

20 g parsley, chopped

Sauté the onion in sesame oil in a wok or saucepan for 5 minutes.

Add the mushrooms, sundried tomatoes, vinegar, red wine and half the parsley.

Mix together thoroughly for 5 minutes, stirring continuously.

Place on a serving platter and sprinkle with the remaining parsley.

Avocado Seafood Starter

(Serves 2–4)

The juice of ½ lemon

4 tablespoons dry white wine

1 teaspoon curry powder

150 g mayonnaise

½ teaspoon mace or nutmeg

225 g prawns, cleaned and deveined

450g crabmeat or lobster meat

1 head romaine lettuce, cleaned and leaves separated

2 avocados, peeled and halved

1 grapefruit, peeled and sectioned

Mix the lemon juice, white wine, curry powder, mayonnaise and nutmeg in a small bowl and set aside.

Place the prawns and crabmeat in a bowl and add half the dressing. Leave to marinade slightly.

Arrange the lettuce leaves to form cups on plates.

Place the avocado halves in the lettuce cups and spoon in the seafood and dressing. Place 4 grapefruit sections on the side of each plate and serve.

Chapter 5:
Mains

Curried Fish

(Serves 4)

900 g sea bass or halibut, bones removed

3 onions, sliced

3 garlic cloves

1 teaspoon cayenne pepper

1 tablespoon curry powder

125 ml white wine vinegar (optional)

½ teaspoon ground cardamom

½ teaspoon cumin

½ teaspoon salt

4 tomatoes

2 tablespoon olive oil

Preheat the oven to 180°C or Gas Mark 4. Place the fish on a baking tray and add the onions over the fish. In a food processor, mix the garlic, pepper, curry, vinegar, cardamom, cumin and salt until smooth. Add the tomatoes and oil, and blend for just 10 seconds. Avoid blending until smooth.

Pour this mixture over the fish. Cover and bake in the oven for 30 minutes or until the fish is cooked. Can be served with whole meal pitta or with rice.

Middle Eastern Couscous

(Serves 4)

450 ml water

1 tablespoon unsalted butter

Grated peel and juice of 1 orange

1 tablespoon honey

½ teaspoon cinnamon

¼ teaspoon nutmeg

¼ teaspoon salt

275 g couscous

110 g almonds, sliced

110 g raisins

110 g dates, chopped

Mix the water, half the butter, orange peel and juice, honey or agave nectar, cinnamon, nutmeg and salt in a medium saucepan and boil.

Add the couscous to the boiling mixture. Then remove from the heat and cover for 10 minutes or until all the liquid has been absorbed.

In a small frying pan, heat the almonds over a medium heat, stirring continuously until they are toasted.

Add the raisins, dates and remaining butter.

Heat until the butter has melted.

Spread the couscous on a serving platter and top with almond and date mixture.

Serve on its own or with grilled chicken or fish.

Fish in a Rich Tomato Sauce

(Serves 4)

1 kg halibut or sea bass (any white fish is fine), cleaned

Salt and pepper to taste

3 tablespoons grape seed oil

1 onion, finely chopped

2½ cm ginger, crushed

3 garlic cloves, crushed

10 g fresh thyme, chopped

225 g tomatoes, crushed

2 tablespoon tomato paste

125 ml dry sherry

25 g fresh parsley, chopped

25 g fresh coriander, chopped

Juice of ½ lemon (optional)

Preheat the oven to 150°C or Gas Mark 2.

Cut the fish into serving slices and then reassemble to make the whole fish again.

Season with salt and pepper to taste.

Place the reassembled fish on a baking tray and bake in the oven for 10–15 minutes.

Remove from the oven and set aside. Heat the oil in a frying pan.

Sauté the onion, ginger, garlic and thyme.

Add the crushed tomatoes and tomato paste and mix well. Add salt and pepper to taste.

Simmer for 10–15 minutes, then gradually add the sherry. Add half the chopped parsley, coriander and lemon juice. Simmer until the sauce thickens to your preferred consistency.

Preheat the oven again to 200°C or Gas Mark 6.

Sprinkle the remaining parsley and coriander on the fish in the baking tray. Pour the tomato sauce over the fish evenly then put the fish back in the oven and bake for 10 minutes.

Reduce the heat to 150°C and bake for a further 5 minutes. Serve hot with fresh bread or boiled or baked yams.

Moroccan Salmon

(Serves 4–6)

350 g green lentils

1½ liters water

¼ teaspoon salt

½ teaspoon freshly ground black pepper

2 tablespoons coriander seeds

2 tablespoons fennel seeds

2 tablespoons cumin seeds

1 teaspoon cardamom seeds

2 teaspoons whole cloves

6 tablespoons grape seed oil

8 garlic cloves, crushed

2 large shallots, chopped

2 tablespoons harissa or any hot sauce

500 g tomatoes, chopped

6 salmon fillets (175 g each with skin)

Place the lentils in a saucepan and cover with water. Bring to the boil over a high heat. Reduce the heat to low, cover and simmer for 25 minutes, stirring occasionally until the lentils are tender. Season with salt and pepper and set aside, covered.

In a frying pan, mix the coriander, fennel, cumin and cardamom seeds with the cloves. Toast the spices over a medium heat for about 3 minutes, stirring until fragrant. Transfer to a plate to cool. Blend the spices in a food processor or with a mortar and pestle.

In a saucepan, heat 4 tablespoon of grape seed oil over a low heat. Sauté the garlic and shallots for 5 minutes. Add the harissa and 1 tablespoon of the spice mixture and cook, stirring for 3 minutes. Add the tomatoes and juices and simmer over a medium heat for 5 minutes, stirring occasionally. Season with salt and pepper to taste.

Preheat the oven to 200°C or Gas Mark. Season the salmon with salt and pepper and coat with the remaining spice mixture on both sides.

Take 2 ovenproof pans and heat 1 tablespoon of oil in each. Add 3 salmon fillets to each pan, skin-side down with a piece of butter next to each fillet and sauté for 3 minutes. Transfer the pans to the oven without turning the salmon and bake for about 6 minutes or until the skins are crisp and the fish is cooked through.

Reheat the lentils and tomato sauce. Spoon lentils onto the center of each dinner plate and place the salmon fillets on top of the lentils. Spoon tomato sauce around the lentils and serve.

Moroccan Chicken Tagine

(Serves 2–4)

2 large onions, chopped

1 whole chicken, cut into small pieces

1 teaspoon black pepper

½ teaspoon turmeric

1 cinnamon stick (use 2 sticks if you want a stronger cinnamon aroma and flavor)

450 ml water

450 g dried apricots

2 teaspoons ground cinnamon

3 tablespoons honey

4 tablespoons grape seed oil

50 g almonds, peeled

1 tablespoon sesame seeds

Sauté the onions in a large saucepan until soft.

Add the chicken, salt, pepper, turmeric, cinnamon stick and water and bring to the boil.

Reduce the heat and simmer for 20 minutes or until the chicken is cooked. Add more water if necessary.

Remove the chicken.

Add the apricots to the saucepan and simmer for 10 minutes.

Add the ground cinnamon and honey or agave.

Stir and simmer until the sauce has slightly thickened.

Add more honey if necessary.

Sauté the almonds in oil for 2 minutes.

Drain the oil from the pan, add the sesame seeds and toast.

Return the chicken to the saucepan to reheat.

To serve, place the chicken on plates.

Pour over the sauce and top with almonds and sesame seeds.

King Prawns in Peanut Sauce

(Serves 2–4)

250g jasmine rice (or any other fragrant rice)

2 red bell peppers, seeds removed

2 red fresh chili peppers

1 onion, chopped

2½ cm ginger, crushed

1 garlic clove

10 ml water

200 g large king prawns

1 tablespoon unsalted peanuts, roasted

10 g fresh thyme, chopped

15 g fresh coriander, chopped

1 chicken stock cube

½ teaspoon salt

½ teaspoon black pepper

1 teaspoon curry powder

Boil the rice using the cooking instructions on the packet.

In a food processor, blend the red peppers, chili, onion, ginger, garlic and water until smooth.

Pour the mixture into a saucepan and simmer on a low heat for 15–20 minutes.

Then add the prawns.

Blend the peanuts and herbs in a food processor.

Add to the sauce and mix well.

Add the chicken stock cube, salt, pepper and the curry powder.

Mix and cook for 10 minutes.

Spoon the rice onto a plate, top with peanut sauce and serve.

Chili Crab with Kale

(Serves 2–4)

1 tablespoon ketchup

125 ml water

1 tablespoon soy sauce

1 tablespoon tomato paste

1 teaspoon corn flour

1 tablespoon sesame oil

2 shallots, chopped

2 garlic cloves, crushed

2½ cm ginger, crushed

1 tablespoon red chili, crushed

200 g baby kale

450 g crabmeat

In a medium bowl, mix the ketchup, water, soy sauce, tomato paste and corn flour. Heat the oil in a saucepan and sauté the shallots for 5 minutes. Add the garlic, ginger and chili and cook for 1 minute.

Add the spinach and cook until just wilted, which takes about 2 minutes. Stir in the sauce and the crabmeat and simmer over a medium heat, stirring occasionally for 5 minutes. Serve with rice.

Wasabi Salmon Burgers

(Serves 2–4)

2 tablespoon soy sauce

1 teaspoon wasabi powder (use more if required)

½ teaspoon honey

450 g salmon fillet, skinned

2 spring onions, chopped

1 egg, lightly beaten

2½ cm ginger, minced

1 teaspoon sesame oil

4 tablespoon grape seed oil

Mix the soy sauce, wasabi powder and honey in a small bowl until smooth. Set aside. Chop the salmon with a large knife into 5 mm pieces and transfer to a bowl. Add the spring onions, egg, and ginger and sesame oil. Mix thoroughly. Form the mixture into 4 burgers. The mixture will be moist and loose, but it holds together when the first side is cooked.

Heat the grape seed oil in a non-stick frying pan over a medium heat. Add the burgers and cook for 5 minutes. Turn and continue to cook until they are firm and fragrant, which takes about 5 minutes. Spoon wasabi sauce evenly over the burgers and cook for a further 30 seconds.

Israeli Couscous

(Serves 4)

225 g couscous

300 ml boiling water

2 carrots, finely chopped

2 celery stalks, finely chopped

1 green pepper, chopped

4 spring onions, chopped

4 sprigs parsley, chopped

50 g raisins

4 tablespoon olive oil

Juice of ½ lemon

1 garlic clove, crushed

½ teaspoon salt

Black pepper

Place the couscous in a medium bowl and add the boiling water. Cover and let stand for about 20 minutes or until the water has been absorbed and the couscous has cooled slightly. Add the finely chopped vegetables, herbs and raisins. In a small bowl, mix the oil, lemon juice, garlic, salt and pepper.

Add the mixture to the salad and toss to blend.

Ginger Fried Rice

(Serves 4–6)

3 teaspoons sesame oil

2 eggs, beaten

6 spring onions, chopped

2½ cm ginger, minced

500 g long-grain brown rice, cooked

150 g frozen peas

100 g mung bean sprouts

2 tablespoon oyster sauce

Heat 1 teaspoon of sesame oil in a wok over a medium heat. Add the eggs and scramble. Transfer to a plate and set aside.

Pour the remaining oil into the wok. Add the spring onions and ginger and stir fry for about 2 minutes until fragrant. Add the rice and peas and stir fry for about 4 minutes until hot and beginning to stick to the wok. Add the bean sprouts, oyster sauce and the eggs. Stir fry, breaking up the eggs for about 2 minutes.

Serve immediately.

Bengali Fish

(Serves 4)

1 kg cod fillets

1 teaspoon turmeric

6 tablespoon mustard oil or grape seed oil

1 teaspoon salt

4 fresh green chilies, chopped

2½ cm ginger, crushed

2 garlic cloves, crushed

2 onions, chopped

2 tomatoes, chopped

425 ml water

15 g fresh coriander, chopped

Preheat the oven to 180°C or Gas Mark 4.

Cut the cod into bite-sized pieces.

In a small bowl, mix the turmeric, half the oil and salt together. Pour over the fish.

Place on a baking tray and bake for 10 minutes.

Remove and set aside.

In a food processor, blend the green chili, ginger, garlic, onions, tomatoes and remaining oil into a paste.

Pour into a saucepan and simmer for 10 minutes.

Remove from the heat and gently place the fish in the sauce without breaking up the fish.

Return the saucepan to a medium heat.

Add the water and cook for 15–20 minutes.

Garnish with coriander and serve.

Indian Lamb Stew

(Serves 4–6)

2 tablespoons grape seed oil

2 onions, chopped

5 garlic cloves

400 g lamb, diced

400 g tomatoes

1 tablespoon cumin

1 teaspoon coriander

½ teaspoon turmeric

¼ teaspoon cayenne pepper

3 teaspoons salt

400 g potatoes, diced

200 g red lentils

700 ml water

Heat the oil in a saucepan and sauté the onion, garlic and lamb for 15 minutes. Add the tomatoes, cumin, coriander, turmeric, pepper and salt. Cook on a high heat for 10–15 minutes.

Add the potatoes, lentils and water. Simmer on a low heat for 1 hour and 10 minutes. Serve when cooked.

Chicken Kadai

(Serves 4)

2 tablespoons grape seed oil

1 onion, chopped

2 garlic cloves, chopped

2½ cm ginger, minced

450 g skinless chicken breast, diced

3 tomatoes, peeled and chopped

1 teaspoon turmeric

2 teaspoons garam masala

½ teaspoon chili powder (or to your taste)

Juice of ½ lemon

1 teaspoon salt

2 teaspoons coriander to garnish

Sauté the onion, garlic and ginger in oil for 10 minutes. Add the chicken, tomatoes, spices, lemon juice and salt. Mix until the chicken is thoroughly coated and sauté for 5 minutes.

Cover and simmer over a low heat for 45 minutes. Garnish with coriander and serve.

Curried Lentils with Sweet Potatoes and Kale

(Serves 4)

1 tablespoon olive oil

1 onion, chopped

2 garlic cloves, crushed

1 tablespoon curry powder

2½ cm ginger, minced

1 teaspoon ground cumin

200 g dried lentils, rinsed

600 ml vegetable or chicken stock

1 sweet potato, peeled and cut into 5 mm cubes

100 g baby kale

Salt and pepper to taste

225 ml plain yoghurt (optional)

50 g almonds, chopped

Heat the oil in a medium saucepan.

Add the onion and garlic and sauté for 5 minutes.

Stir in the curry powder, ginger and cumin and cook for 1 minute.

Add the lentils and stock and bring to the boil. Reduce the heat and simmer, covered, for 10 minutes.

Add the sweet potato, cover and cook for 10 minutes until soft.

Stir in the spinach and cook for 1 minute until the spinach is just wilted. Add salt and pepper to taste.

Transfer to bowls and top each with 1 tablespoon of yoghurt and 1 tablespoon of chopped almonds.

Serve hot.

Salmon in a Spicy Tomato Sauce

(Serves 2–4)

2 teaspoon olive oil

1 onion, coarsely chopped

2 garlic cloves, chopped

1 red bell pepper, chopped

2 tomatoes, coarsely chopped

15 g fresh coriander, chopped

1 can tomatoes, diced

2 tablespoons paprika

1 tablespoon ground cumin

2 teaspoons salt

2 tablespoons cayenne pepper

1 teaspoon ground black pepper

125 ml water

450g salmon fillets, cut into 4 individual slices

Juice of ½ lemon

Preheat the oven to 180°C or Gas Mark 4.

Heat the oil in an ovenproof frying pan and sauté the onion and garlic for 5 minutes.

Add the red pepper, chopped fresh tomatoes and coriander. Sauté until tender.

In a medium bowl, mix the canned diced tomatoes, 1 tablespoon paprika, cumin, salt, 1 tablespoon cayenne pepper, ground black pepper and water together thoroughly.

Add half the mixture to the pan and cook for 10 minutes.

Sprinkle 1 tablespoon paprika and 1 tablespoon cayenne onto the salmon and rub in.

Add the salmon to the sauce and cook for 10 minutes.

Pour the remaining tomato mixture over the salmon and continue to cook for another 10 minutes.

Add the lemon juice, cover and cook for 5 minutes or until salmon is cooked through. Remove the cover and place the pan in the oven.

Broil for 7 minutes and then serve.

Saffron, Courgettes, Peppers and Herb Couscous

(Serves 4)

300 ml chicken stock

1 teaspoon salt

½ teaspoon fresh ground black pepper

¼ teaspoon ground cumin

½ teaspoon saffron threads

1 tablespoon olive oil

1 tablespoon unsalted butter

2 courgettes, diced

1 onion, chopped

1 red bell pepper, chopped

1 green bell pepper, chopped

250 g couscous

25 g fresh basil, chopped

25 g fresh parsley, chopped

Boil the chicken stock in a saucepan and then turn off the heat.

Add the salt, pepper, cumin and saffron threads and allow to steep for at least 15 minutes.

Heat the olive oil and butter in a saucepan.

Add the courgettes, onion, red and green peppers, and cook for 5 minutes or until lightly browned.

Bring the stock back to the boil.

Place the couscous in a large bowl, add the courgettes and peppers and pour into the hot chicken stock.

Cover the bowl tightly with a cover or cling film and leave to stand for 15 minutes.

Add the basil and parsley.

Using a fork, toss the couscous and herbs.

Serve warm.

Curried Mussels and Tomato

(Serves 4)

1 tablespoon grape seed oil

2½ cm ginger, chopped

2 garlic cloves, crushed

1 sprig fresh curry leaves

1 can plum tomatoes

½ teaspoon chili powder

½ teaspoon turmeric

½ teaspoon tamarind paste

200 ml water

½ teaspoon cumin seeds

½ teaspoon salt

½ teaspoon honey

2 kg fresh mussels

1 sprig fresh mint, finely chopped

10 g bean sprouts

1 red chili, seeds removed, chopped

1 sprig fresh coriander, finely chopped

Heat the oil in a large saucepan and sauté the ginger and garlic.

Add the curry leaves, tomatoes, chili powder, turmeric and tamarind.

Cook for 2 minutes.

Pour in the water and simmer for 10 minutes.

Crush the cumin seeds and add to the sauce.

Strain the sauce through a sieve.

Add the salt and honey.

Put the mussels in the sauce and simmer for 3 minutes until they open.

Discard any that haven't opened. Place in bowls.

Garnish with mint, bean sprouts, red chilies and coriander and serve.

Halibut with Mediterranean Salsa

(Serves 2–4)

4 halibut fillets

2 tablespoon water

½ teaspoon chili powder

1 teaspoon dried thyme

1 teaspoon freshly grated lemon zest

1 tomato, deseeded and chopped

1 (60g) can Kalamata olives or ripe olives, drained and sliced

15 g fresh parsley, chopped

Juice of ½ lemon

1 tablespoon capers, drained (optional)

2 teaspoons extra virgin olive oil

1 teaspoon dried oregano

Preheat the oven to 160°C or Gas Mark 3.

Coat a baking dish with cooking oil spray and arrange the fish in a single layer.

Pour the water over the fish and sprinkle with chili powder, thyme and lemon zest.

Cover the dish with foil and bake for 15 minutes.

In a small bowl, mix the tomato, olives, parsley, lemon juice, capers, oil and oregano thoroughly.

Place the fish on a serving platter, top with the salsa and serve.

Tofu with Tomatoes and Coriander

(Serves 4)

1 tablespoon grape seed oil

6 spring onions, chopped

2 garlic cloves, crushed

3 tomatoes, deseeded and cut into 2½ cm squares

450 g fresh extra firm tofu, drained and cut into 2½ cm squares

1 teaspoon salt (optional)

½ teaspoon honey

1 teaspoon soy sauce

¼ teaspoon ground coriander

½ teaspoon black pepper

Heat the oil in a wok or saucepan.

Stir fry the spring onions and garlic for 2 minutes.

Add the tomatoes and stir fry for 1 minute.

Add the tofu, salt, honey, soy sauce and coriander.

Stir to blend in and cook for 30 seconds.

Season with black pepper and serve hot.

Spicy Mackerel

(Serves 4–6)

8 mackerel fillets

½ teaspoon salt

Juice of ½ lime

1 tablespoon grapeseed oil

2 carrots, grated

½ teaspoon ground coriander

½ teaspoon ground cumin

½ teaspoon aniseed

1 teaspoon chili powder

Preheat the oven to 180°C or Gas Mark 4.

Line an oven tray with foil and grease the foil.

Put the fillets on the tray skin-side down.

Rub in the salt and pour over the lime juice.

Brush with half the oil and bake for about 5 minutes.

Mix the remaining oil, carrots, coriander, cumin, aniseed and chili.

Sprinkle the mixture over the fish and grill for 2 minutes.

Mediterranean Rice and Beans

(Serves 4)

2 tablespoons olive oil

1 onion, finely chopped

1 garlic clove, crushed

225 g basmati rice, uncooked and washed

2 teaspoons ground cumin

2 teaspoons ground coriander

1 teaspoon turmeric

1 teaspoon cayenne pepper

1 liter vegetable stock

675 g minced lamb

1 (400g) can chickpeas, drained and rinsed

1 (400g) can black beans, drained and rinsed

Juice of 1 lemon

30 g fresh coriander, chopped

15 g fresh parsley, chopped

4 tablespoons pine nuts

½ teaspoon salt

½ teaspoon ground black pepper

Heat 1 tablespoon of the olive oil in a medium saucepan.

Sauté the onion and garlic for 5 minutes.

Add the rice, cumin, coriander, turmeric and cayenne pepper.

Cook, stirring constantly for 7 minutes.

Add the vegetable stock and bring to the boil.

Reduce the heat, cover and simmer for 20 minutes.

Sauté the lamb in the remaining olive oil in a saucepan over a medium heat until it is evenly browned.

Mix the lamb, chickpeas, black beans, lemon juice, coriander, parsley and pine nuts with the cooked rice.

Add salt and pepper to taste.

Serve.

Chicken in Spicy Tomato and Herb Sauce

(Serves 4)

4 chicken breasts, cut in half

1 tablespoon salt

Juice of ½ lemon

5 garlic cloves, roughly chopped

2½ cm ginger, roughly chopped

2 onions, chopped

4 tablespoons grapeseed oil

1 cinnamon stick, halved

4 green cardamom pods, bruised

4 cloves

1 teaspoon chili powder

½ teaspoon turmeric

1 tablespoon ground coriander

250g can chopped tomatoes

1 tablespoon black peppercorns, coarsely crushed

240 ml warm water

Rub the lemon juice and salt into the chicken and set aside.

In a food processor, blend the garlic, ginger and onions until smooth.

Heat the oil in a large saucepan.

Add the cinnamon, cardamom and cloves.

Let the spices sizzle gently until the cardamom pods plump up.

Add the blended ingredients and stir fry over a medium heat for 5–6 minutes.

Reduce the heat and continue stir frying for a further 4 minutes.

Add the chili powder, turmeric, coriander and tomatoes.

Cook over a medium heat for 5–6 minutes stirring regularly.

Add the black pepper and chicken.

Cook over a high heat for about 5 minutes. Pour in the water and bring to the boil. Then reduce the heat, cover and simmer for 25 minutes.

Remove the lid and cook for a further 6–8 minutes, until the sauce has reduced to a thick paste.

Serve with basmati rice.

Portuguese Rice and Sausage

(Serves 4–6)

300 g basmati rice

8 Portuguese sausages, cut into thick slices

4 tablespoons grape seed oil

1 cinnamon stick

6 green cardamom pods, bruised

6 cloves

1 onion, halved and sliced

3 garlic cloves, crushed

1 teaspoon chili powder

½ teaspoon turmeric

1 green chili, deseeded and chopped

½ teaspoon salt

500 ml warm water

Wash the rice several times in cold water until clear, then leave to soak in fresh water for 15 minutes.

Grill the sausages until browned and cooked through.

Heat the oil in a saucepan over a low heat.

Add the cinnamon, cardamom and cloves, and let them sizzle until the cardamom pods are plumped up.

Add the onion and cook for about 8 minutes until browned.

Add the garlic, chili powder, turmeric and green chili. Cook for 2–3 minutes.

Drain the rice and add it to the saucepan.

Stir over a medium heat for 2 minutes then add the salt and pour in the water.

Bring to the boil over a high heat. Reduce the heat to medium and cook uncovered for 10–15 minutes until the water has been absorbed.

Reduce the heat further to low, mix in the sausages, cover and cook for 6 minutes.

Turn the heat off and leave to stand for about 10 minutes before serving.

Split Peas with Mango Salsa

(Serves 4)

560 ml water

225 g yellow split peas, rinsed and drained

1 mango, peeled and cubed

110 ml salsa

100 g can pineapple chunks, chopped coarsely

10 g coriander, chopped

2 teaspoon white wine vinegar

Juice of ½ lime

½ teaspoon ground cumin

2 tablespoon olive oil

5 spring onions, chopped

½ teaspoon powdered ginger

½ teaspoon ground allspice

¼ teaspoon ground cardamom

Juice of ½ orange

4 tablespoon vegetable stock

½ teaspoon honey

200 g kale, washed and chopped

Put the split peas and water in a medium saucepan and bring to the boil over a medium heat.

Reduce the heat to low, cover and simmer for 30 minutes or until tender.

Drain and set aside.

In a medium bowl, mix the mango, salsa, pineapple, coriander, vinegar, lime juice and cumin together. Set aside.

Heat 1 tablespoon of the oil in a large non-stick frying pan.

Add the spring onions and sauté, stirring for 3 minutes.

Add the ginger, allspice and cardamom and cook for a minute.

Stir in the orange juice, stock and honey.

Add the split peas and cook, stirring frequently for 10–15 minutes or until the mixture thickens.

In another saucepan, heat the remaining oil, add the kale and cook, stirring constantly for 4–5 minutes or until the kale is just wilted.

Place the kale on a serving platter, top with the split peas mixture, then with the mango mixture and serve.

Vegetable Casserole

(Serves 4)

Peel and juice of 1 orange

2 teaspoons corn flour

6 sweet potatoes, cut into cubes

2 onions, cut into 6 wedges

2 leeks, thickly sliced

2 carrots, peeled and sliced into 1 cm thick rounds

150 g pitted prunes, halved

525g can unsweetened pineapple chunks

1 cm ginger, chopped

1 teaspoon ground cinnamon

4 tablespoons toasted almonds, chopped

Preheat the oven to 190°C or Gas Mark 5. Coat a baking dish with non-stick spray. In a large bowl, mix the orange juice and corn flour until smooth.

Add the orange peel, sweet potatoes, onions, leeks, carrots, and prunes, pineapple chunks with juice, ginger and cinnamon. Mix well to blend, pour into the baking dish and cover with foil. Bake in the oven for 45 minutes. Remove the foil and sprinkle with almonds. Bake for another 15 minutes and serve.

Greek Stuffed Tomatoes

(Serves 3–6)

2 tablespoons olive oil

1 onion, chopped

100 g kale, chopped

Handful of parsley, chopped

2 teaspoon dried basil

½ teaspoon crushed chili (optional)

50 g breadcrumbs

225 g feta cheese, crumbled

½ teaspoon salt

½ teaspoon black pepper

6 large tomatoes, firm and insides scooped out

Preheat the oven to 180°C or Gas Mark 4. Heat the oil in a saucepan over a medium heat and sauté the onion for 5 minutes. Add the spinach and cook for 2 minutes.

In a bowl, mix the onion, spinach, parsley, basil, crushed chili, breadcrumbs, cheese, salt and pepper together. Stuff the mixture into the tomatoes and bake for 15 minutes. Serve.

Seafood Stew

(Serves 4)

4 tablespoons olive oil

1 onion, chopped

3 celery stalks, chopped

1 green & 1 red bell pepper, chopped

5 garlic cloves, crushed

½ teaspoon red pepper, crushed

2 teaspoons dried oregano

1 teaspoon dried marjoram

3 tablespoons fresh basil, chopped

450 ml bottled clam juice

2 cans (425 g) chopped tomatoes

140 ml red wine

450 g white fish, cubed (halibut, haddock or cod)

450g king prawns, shelled and deveined

450 g scallops (washed and cut in half) or mussels (pre-cooked, removed from shells and cut in half)

Juice of ½ lemon

½ teaspoon salt and coarsely ground black pepper

Grated parmesan cheese to garnish

Heat the oil in a medium saucepan over a medium heat.

Add the onion and sauté for 5 minutes.

Add the celery and peppers and sauté for 2 minutes.

Stir in the garlic, crushed pepper, oregano, marjoram and basil.

Lower the heat and cook for 2 minutes.

Add the clam juice, tomatoes and wine.

Cover and simmer for 15 minutes.

Add the fish, prawns, scallops or mussels.

Cook for 4–5 minutes or until the seafood is just cooked.

Stir in the lemon juice and season with salt and pepper to taste.

Garnish with grated parmesan.

Ratatouille

(Serves 4)

4 tablespoons olive oil

1 onion, chopped

5 garlic cloves, crushed

1 bay leaf

1 eggplant, washed and cubed

1 teaspoon salt

15 g fresh basil, chopped

2 teaspoons dried oregano

1 teaspoon rosemary

2 courgettes, washed and cubed

2 yellow squash, washed and cubed

1 red bell pepper, deseeded and chopped

1 green bell pepper, deseeded and chopped

3 tomatoes, chopped

125 ml dry red wine

225 g mushrooms, sliced

15 g fresh parsley, chopped

2 tablespoon parmesan cheese, grated (optional)

Heat the olive oil in a saucepan.

Add the onion, garlic and bay leaf, and sauté for 5 minutes.

Add the eggplant, salt, basil, oregano and rosemary.

Cover and cook over a medium heat for 10 minutes, stirring occasionally.

Add the courgettes, yellow squash, peppers, tomatoes and wine.

Cover and simmer over a low heat for 10 minutes.

Mix in the mushrooms and parsley.

Simmer for 5 minutes or until the vegetables are tender.

Remove the bay leaf.

Serve on a plate and garnish with parmesan.

Chapter 6:
Desserts

Creamy Dark Chocolate and Almond Mousse

(Serves 4)

75 ml water

1 teaspoon almond extract

2 tablespoons honey

125 g dark chocolate powder (more than 70 percent cocoa)

2 avocados, deseeded and peeled

2 tablespoons almonds, crushed

1 sprig mint (garnish)

In a food processor, blend the water, almond extract, honey or agave nectar, chocolate and avocados until smooth.

Spoon into goblets or ice cream bowls and refrigerate for an hour or until ready to serve.

Sprinkle with crushed almonds and garnish with 1 mint leaf per serving.

Coconut Candy

(Serves 6–8)

 4 tablespoons honey

 2 coconuts, flesh shredded (or 700 g dried coconut)

2 tablespoons water

In a saucepan, heat the honey.

Mix the coconut and water in a bowl and add to the saucepan.

Cook for about 5 minutes, stirring continuously.

Remove from the heat and allow to cool a little.

Scoop 1 or 2 tablespoons into the palm of your hand and roll into a ball.

Place on a platter and repeat using all the mixture.

Allow to cool completely and harden.

Baked Bananas

(Serves 6–8)

4 tablespoons fresh orange juice

1 tablespoon flour

2 tablespoons honey

3 tablespoons cinnamon

8 bananas, cut diagonally into 3 pieces

250 ml sour cream

110 g coconut, shredded

Preheat the oven to 180°C or Gas Mark 4.

In a small bowl, mix the orange juice, flour, honey or agave and half the cinnamon until smooth.

Place the bananas in an ovenproof dish and glaze with the syrup.

Cover with foil and bake for 10 minutes.

Place a piece of banana in each individual compote dish and top with 3 tablespoon of sour cream.

Dust with cinnamon and sprinkle with 1 tablespoon of coconut.

Fruit Salad

(Serves 4–6)

½ melon, cubed

2 apples, cored and cubed

2 bananas, sliced

5 oranges, peeled, deseeded and chopped

Juice of 3 oranges

Juice of 1 lemon

1½ tablespoon honey

1 teaspoon vanilla essence

1 teaspoon cinnamon

Mix all the ingredients in a large bowl.
Chill before serving.

Mango and Banana Sundae

(Serves 2–4)

1 mango, peeled and chopped

2 bananas, peeled and chopped

Juice of ½ lemon

Juice of 2 oranges

Vanilla ice cream

In a medium bowl, mix the mango, bananas, lemon juice and orange juice together.

Spoon the fruit salad into ice cream bowls, top with a scoop of ice cream and serve.

Watermelon with Fennel Seeds

This is a really great soothing dessert after a large, rich meal – the fennel soothes indigestion and the watermelon is light and tasty.

(Serves 4–6)

1 tablespoon fennel seeds

2 teaspoons salt

1 watermelon, quartered and cut into 2½ cm thick slices

2 limes, cut into wedges

Heat a frying pan over a low heat for about 3 minutes until hot.

Add the fennel seeds and toast, stirring constantly for 3–4 minutes.

Transfer to a plate and allow to cool.

In a food processor or using a mortar and pestle, crush the fennel seeds.

Mix the seeds with salt and sprinkle over the watermelon.

Serve with lime wedges.

Green Tea Poached Pears with Cream

(Serves 4)

850 ml water

1½ tablespoons green tea leaves

3 tablespoons honey

1 tablespoon crystallized ginger, chopped

½ teaspoon almond extract

4 firm, ripe pears, halved and cored

1 tablespoon sliced almonds, toasted

125 ml single cream

Bring the water to the boil in a saucepan. Add the green tea leaves and stir. Turn off the heat and cover, allowing to steep for 5 minutes. Pour through a sieve into a bowl to remove the leaves and return to the saucepan. Add the honey, ginger and almond extract, and bring to the boil. Add the pears, cut side up, and poach over a low heat until quite tender when pierced with a fork. Transfer to a bowl and let the pears cool in the liquid. Chill for 30 minutes.

Place 2 pear halves in each dessert dish. Pour 2 tablespoon of sauce over the pears, top with 2 tablespoon of cream and garnish with almonds.

Spiced Dried Fruit Compote

(Serves 2–4)

225 ml water

1 green teabag

175 g dried apricots, halved

110 g dried figs, halved

110 g dried cherries

1 tablespoon honey

1 cm ginger

1 strip lemon rind

1 small cinnamon stick

In a medium saucepan, bring the water to the boil and then remove from the heat.

Add the teabag and allow to steep for 5 minutes.

Remove and discard the bag. Add the apricots, figs, cherries, honey, ginger, lemon rind and cinnamon stick. Bring to the boil. Reduce the heat to low and simmer, stirring occasionally, for 15–20 minutes or until the fruit is tender.

Remove and discard the ginger, lemon rind and cinnamon stick. Serve warm or chilled.

Pears in Red Wine

(Serves 4)

4 firm pears, washed and peeled, saving the skin

500 ml red wine

2 tablespoons agave nectar or unrefined brown sugar

1 cinnamon stick

Cream or ice cream (optional)

Place the pears and skins in a large saucepan and add the wine, agave or sugar and the cinnamon. Bring to the boil over a medium heat for about 20 minutes, turning the pears over. Remove the pears from the liquid, place in a dish and set aside.

Continue cooking the red wine with the skins and cinnamon, slowly reducing the liquid until all the alcohol has evaporated and the liquid consistency is thick.

Remove the cinnamon and pear skins from the syrup and cook further for 5 minutes. Add the pears to the syrup and cook for 5 minutes. Turn off the heat and let the pears cool to room temperature.

Place in individual dessert bowls and top with syrup.

Serve plain or with ice cream or cream.

Spiced Oranges

(Serves 4–6)

4 tablespoons honey (or 2 tablespoon unrefined brown sugar)

2 cloves

1 cinnamon stick

1 cm ginger, sliced thinly

500 ml carton orange juice

6 oranges, peeled, pith and pips removed, and sliced thinly

Fresh cream to serve

Toasted flaked almonds

Place all the ingredients in a saucepan except the sliced oranges, cream and flaked almonds.

Bring to a boil and simmer on a low heat for 1½ hours, stirring occasionally, or until the mixture thickens like syrup.

Mix in the orange slices and transfer to a bowl. Serve in dessert bowls.

Top each with 1 tablespoon of cream and sprinkle with 1 tablespoon of flaked almonds.

Chapter 7:
Smoothie Recipes

Cleanse Smoothie

(Serves 1)

100g baby kale, washed

Juice of 1 lemon

Juice of 1 lime

1 cucumber

3 celery sticks

1 apple

1 cm ginger

1 kiwi, peeled (optional)

½ avocado (optional)

½ teaspoon honey (optional)

Put all ingredients except the honey into your blender and blend until smooth.

Add the honey if required.

Add ice cubes and crush for a more refreshing smoothie.

Peach and Mint Smoothie

(Serves 1)

100g baby kale, washed

2 peaches, peeled, cored and cubed

3 sprigs mint, washed

1 apple, peeled, cored and cubed

Juice of ½ lemon

½ cucumber, peeled if not organic

1 teaspoon honey

Place all ingredients in a blender and blend until smooth.

It tastes even better with crushed ice.

Antioxidant Boost

(Serves 1)

75g blueberries, washed

75g raspberries, washed

1 banana, peeled and chopped

10 strawberries, stems removed and washed

Juice of 1 orange

50 g pomegranate (½ pomegranate with fruit squeezed out)

½ teaspoon honey (optional)

Place all ingredients in a blender and blend until smooth.

Pineapple Blast

(Serves 1)

1 pineapple, peeled and chopped

Juice of 1 lemon

2½ cm ginger

1 tablespoon Manuka honey

Blend all ingredients in a blender or juicer.

Super-Charged Cinnamon

(Serves 1)

½ blender of almond or rice milk

75g berries (blueberries, cherries or raspberries)

1 avocado

1 banana

3 heaped tablespoon fresh bee pollen

1 tablespoon raw, organic honey

4 tablespoon ground sprouted flax powder

1 teaspoon cinnamon

Half fill your blender with the almond or rice milk.

Add all the ingredients except for the flax powder and cinnamon.

Turn the blender on low until the mixture is smooth.

Add the flax powder and cinnamon and blend well on high for 2 minutes until creamy.

Power Punch Smoothie

(Serves 1)

½ bunch of celery

1 bag of kale

½ green pepper

½ cucumber

 30 g parsley, chopped

1 avocado

1 scoop alfalfa

1 scoop bean sprouts

4 tablespoons fresh coriander, chopped

1 small tomato

2 spring onions, chopped (optional)

80 ml water, 6 ice cubes

Place all the ingredients in a blender, one by one, and blend until creamy smooth. Add the ice cubes last.

Alternatively, you can make this in a saucepan on your hob using a low temperature. Stir constantly as if you are making a soup.

Leave out the ice cubes to make a warm smoothie.

Chapter 8:

Your Cheat Sheet – Keeping Your Kitchen Well Stocked with Super Foods

The key to success with the recipes in this book is to use the best quality and freshest produce that you can afford. If you can, grow your own veggies – this is the best way to ensure freshness. If that is not an option, see if you can find a local farmer's market and source veggies there once a week. (Just remember to get there early, preferably as it opens so that you get first dibs on the best produce.)

I also do not want you to view the recipes as if written in stone – if you are battling to get a certain ingredient, or you really do not like a particular ingredient, feel free to swap it out and use something else. Experimenting and making the recipe your own is one of the really fun aspects about cooking – it is not like baking where everything has to be carefully weighed and measured or you risk a complete disaster.

Also consider cooking double quantities of the recipes that you can freeze and freeze half. That way, when you are really rushed for time or really do not feel like cooking, you have your own supply of convenience foods in the freezer waiting for you.

Make it as easy as possible to include these foods by making sure that you have them on hand. It may take a bit more effort to cook a meal from scratch but this is a fair trade off when you consider all the health benefits.

I would just like to add a quick note on convenience foods here. It may be tempting to buy those pre-peeled and chopped vegetables at the grocery store but you really should do your own prep – as soon as the food is prepped, it starts losing nutrients through oxidization and you really have no idea how long that pre-cut stuff has been sitting there. Even more worrying, some of it is soaked in a solution of chlorine so that it has a longer shelf-life – scary, isn't it?

If you want to go the convenience route, buy frozen pre-cut vegetables or fruit instead. These are second only to freshly picked foods as they are quick frozen shortly after they have been picked and so contain a comparable level of nutrients.

Let's go through the basic staples that you should consider having you kitchen cupboard.

Fruits

As far as fruits go, you can choose whichever fruits you prefer. I do suggest using fruits that are in season as far as possible, the fresher the better. Fruit that is out of season is likely to have been subjected to a long cold storage process and was, more than likely, picked before it was optimally ripe. It also tends to be a lot more expensive.

Here are some fruits to consider:

Apples: Vitamin A, C, D, iron, Calcium and magnesium.

Bananas: One of the most common ingredients in the smoothie world. Use to give a great creamy texture and sweet flavor to your smoothie.

Blueberries: Flavorful and chock-full of antioxidants.

Dates: Sweet and full of amino acids and fiber. Pears – Antioxidant.

Goji berries: Aids in well-being, quality of sleep and weight control.

Kiwi fruit: Loaded with Vitamin C.

Mangos: Vitamin C, A, B6, GABA and lots of fiber.

Papaya: Vitamin C, D, B6 and A, along with iron, magnesium and calcium.

Pineapple: Vitamin C, A and B complex, along with manganese and copper.

Raspberries: Antioxidant and anti-inflammatory.

Strawberries: Vitamin C and plenty of minerals. **Oranges**: Vitamin C and fiber.

Greens

These greens are considered Superfoods, along with many of the fruits listed above. Superfoods are simply 'Exceptional" foods that have exceptional nutritional properties, which are thought to be highly beneficial for our health.

Kale: Has Vitamin C and A and some important flavonoids.

Spinach: Vitamin K, C, Beta-carotene, iron, magnesium, calcium and protein.

Swiss Chard: Vitamin E and C and is an antioxidant. Dandelion greens – Vitamin C, B6, potassium, calcium and iron. Cilantro – Tasty and is a detoxifier.

Bok Choy: Vitamin A, C, K, magnesium, potassium, manganese, calcium and iron.

Mint leaves: Refreshing and antioxidant, giving energy and soothing digestive upsets.

Nuts Seeds and Other Essentials

All you need is 75g of nuts a day to see the benefits. Eat them over and above your normal protein intake and you'll get a healthy boost. They are calorie dense but it should be remembered that they contain loads of nutrients and monounsaturated fats. Nuts will also help you feel full, give you an energy boost and keep your blood levels more stable.

Almonds: full of protein and fiber and great for boosting energy and satiating hunger. **Cashews**: Low fat and high in minerals.

Walnuts: Vitamin E, flavonoids and is good for the heart.

Chia seeds: Low calorie, high in fiber, protein and minerals.

Flaxseeds: Antioxidant and high in fiber.

Pumpkin seeds: High in Omega-3 fatty acids and a range of nutrients

Sweeteners

I have included a lot of recipes that have honey in them as a sweetener. You can, if you like, switch out the honey for an alternative sweetener such as agave syrup, stevia or xylitol.

Honey or stevia are the best out of the lot of options and they are what I prefer. Watch out when adding stevia because it is a lot sweeter than sugar.

There is just one rule when it comes to sweeteners – no refined sugar of any kind and no artificial sweeteners of any kind.

Refined Sugar is Out

I cannot emphasize how important this is. Refined sugar has no nutrient value at all and will wreak havoc with your body. Even worse, the reason that it tastes so good is that it acts on the pleasure center of the brain, causing a release of endorphins.

It actually has a similar effect on the brain that drugs such as cocaine and heroin do and is just as addictive.

And the real problem – it is in just about everything that you eat. There is no denying it – it really does make food taste better and so is added to just about everything, even foods that you would never dream of in a million years. For example, peanut butter usually contains a lot of sugar and bacon is cured in sugar. And that low-fat fruit yoghurt that is so good for you probably contains the same amount of sugar as a can of soda.

Fortunately, with you preparing your meals from scratch, you can control exactly what goes into them and you can be sure that you are not taking in a whole heap of hidden sugars.

It also does not take too long to get over the sugar cravings – contrary to what you may think, the more sugar you eat, the more you want. As you start to phase it out of your diet, you will find that you crave it less and less.

Conclusion

Thank you again for downloading this book!

I hope that you have found a lot of recipes that you want to try out and I do hope that you enjoy them.

Please consider this book as an introduction into this exciting world and use it as a basis to build your superfood cooking skills in future. I encourage you to read more on superfoods and to learn more about them as you go along. If you enjoyed this book, check out my Superfood Smoothies book on Amazon – or watch out for my soon-to-be-released series on individual superfoods!

Science is discovering new beneficial properties in the foods that we eat all the time so keep reading up on super foods to keep abreast of the latest developments.

All that is left now is to practice what you have learned in this book and to start using the recipes in your daily life!

Finally, I would really appreciate it if you would review this book on Amazon for me. I would love to read your thoughts and it will help me to continue helping people find happiness.

Thank you and good luck!

Printed in Great Britain
by Amazon